About the NCCN Guidelines for Patients®

National Comprehensive Cancer Network®

Did you know that top cancer centers across the United States work together to improve cancer care? This alliance of leading cancer centers is called the National Comprehensive Cancer Network® (NCCN®).

Cancer care is always changing. NCCN develops evidence-based cancer care recommendations used by health care providers worldwide. These frequently updated recommendations are the NCCN Clinical Practice Guidelines in Oncology (NCCN Guidelines®). The NCCN Guidelines for Patients plainly explain these expert recommendations for people with cancer and caregivers.

These NCCN Guidelines for Patients are based on the NCCN Clinical Practice Guidelines in Oncology (NCCN Guidelines®) for Waldenström Macroglobulinemia/Lymphoplasmacytic Lymphoma, Version 3.2025 — February 6, 2025.

Learn how the NCCN Guidelines for Patients are developed
NCCN.org/patient-guidelines-process

View the NCCN Guidelines for Patients free online
NCCN.org/patientguidelines

Find an NCCN Cancer Center near you
NCCN.org/cancercenters

Connect with us

Supporters

NCCN Guidelines for Patients are supported by funding from the NCCN Foundation®

NCCN Foundation gratefully acknowledges the following corporate supporters for helping to make available these NCCN Guidelines for Patients: BeOne Medicines USA, Inc.

NCCN independently adapts, updates, and hosts the NCCN Guidelines for Patients. Our corporate supporters do not participate in the development of the NCCN Guidelines for Patients and are not responsible for the content and recommendations contained therein.

To make a gift or learn more, visit online or email

NCCNFoundation.org/donate

PatientGuidelines@NCCN.org

Contents

NCCN Foundation seeks to support the millions of patients and their families affected by a cancer diagnosis by funding and distributing NCCN Guidelines for Patients. NCCN Foundation is also committed to advancing cancer treatment by funding the nation's promising doctors at the center of innovation in cancer research. For more details and the full library of patient and caregiver resources, visit NCCN.org/patients.

National Comprehensive Cancer Network (NCCN) and NCCN Foundation
3025 Chemical Road, Suite 100, Plymouth Meeting, PA 19462 USA

1

About Waldenström macroglobulinemia

Waldenström macroglobulinemia (WM) is a slow-growing blood cancer that doesn't always require treatment. If treatment is needed, new therapies are giving people more years to live with fewer symptoms.

What is WM?

Waldenström macroglobulinemia (also just called Waldenström) is a rare, slow-growing cancer that affects blood cells. Because WM grows slowly, people with this disease have time to consider their options for treatment and decide when treatment, if needed, should begin.

Treatment for WM mainly involves reducing symptoms. Many effective therapies are available for treating these symptoms.

However, not everyone with Waldenström has symptoms. Some people go without symptoms for many years. People with WM who don't have symptoms don't need treatment.

Importantly, many people with Waldenström can expect to live a normal life span.

Why you should read this book

Making decisions about cancer care can be stressful. You may need to make tough decisions under pressure about complex choices.

The NCCN Guidelines for Patients are trusted by patients and providers. They clearly explain current care recommendations made by respected experts in the field. Recommendations are based on the latest research and practices at leading cancer centers.

Cancer care is not the same for everyone. By following expert recommendations for your situation, you are more likely to improve your care and have better outcomes as a result. Use this book as your guide to find the information you need to make important decisions.

What causes WM?

As with many cancers, researchers aren't sure what causes some people to develop WM.

Waldenström begins in white blood cells called lymphocytes. Lymphocytes are part of the body's immune system. They protect the body from infection by evolving into plasma cells. Plasma cells fight infection by making antibodies. Antibodies are proteins that attack bacteria, viruses, and other harmful substances. Antibodies are also called immunoglobulins. There are 5 main types of immunoglobulins ("Ig" for short): IgA, IgD, IgE, IgG, and IgM.

In WM, something goes wrong with this process: A single immune cell develops a genetic change and grows into a unique cancer made of abnormal lymphocytes, plasma cells, and lymphoplasmacytic cells (a cell that's a cross between a lymphocyte and a plasma cell). Together, these are called WM cells.

WM cells don't behave like normal immune cells. They multiply out of control and crowd out normal blood cells in the bone marrow (the space inside bones where new blood cells are created).

WM cells eventually take over the bone marrow, preventing it from working properly and hindering it from making the blood cells that the body needs. This shortage of blood cells starts to cause health issues that you can feel (symptoms).

WM cells can also build up in other parts of the body, causing swelling and discomfort in areas like the lymph nodes (glands), liver, and spleen.

But who was Waldenström? And what is macroglobulinemia?

Waldenström was Jan Waldenström, a doctor in Sweden who first identified this cancer. **Macroglobulinemia** refers to a large protein that causes a blood condition.

- **"macro"** = large
- **"globulin"** = protein
- **"-emia"** = blood condition

In WM, this large protein is immunoglobulin M (IgM), the largest of the 5 immunoglobulins. It's the only immunoglobulin (antibody) that WM cells make, and they make it in large numbers.

Because WM cells are abnormal, the IgM antibodies they make are also abnormal. First, these IgMs are all identical copies of one another. Second, unlike normal antibodies that fight infection, abnormal IgM antibodies don't help your body and sometimes cause harm.

IgM is the largest antibody

Antibodies are proteins that attack bacteria, viruses, and other harmful substances. Antibodies are also called immunoglobulins (Ig).

The IgM antibody is much larger than the others because it's made up of 5 antibodies, called a pentamer. IgM's bulky size and structure contribute to the abnormal thickening of the blood (hyperviscosity) that occurs in some people with WM.

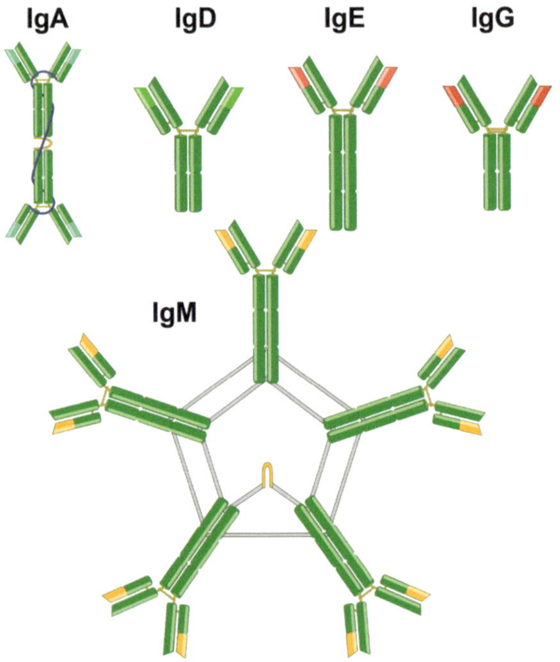

What's more, when these large proteins build up in blood, the blood can thicken—a condition called hyperviscosity syndrome. Thickened blood slows normal blood flow, causing a number of symptoms in the body. It's one of the main signs of WM.

Is there a cure for WM?

Although there's currently no cure for WM, there are many effective therapies that can keep the disease under control, reduce or eliminate symptoms, and improve your quality of life. Controlling problems like hyperviscosity syndrome can be life-saving.

Treatments for WM include targeted therapy, chemotherapy, or a combination of these treatments. For many people, treatment may get Waldenström under control for several years. During this time, most people have no symptoms of the disease.

But even with treatment, WM usually comes back eventually and needs more or different treatment.

Is Waldenström the same as lymphoplasmacytic lymphoma?

The terms Waldenström macroglobulinemia and lymphoplasmacytic lymphoma are often used interchangeably. But they're not exactly the same thing.

Lymphoplasmacytic lymphoma is the cancer, and WM is one type of it. However, WM is by far the most common type of it. Almost everyone who has lymphoplasmacytic lymphoma has WM.

The main difference is that WM has high levels of IgM antibodies, while the other types of lymphoplasmacytic lymphoma are usually linked with IgG or IgA antibodies. Still, treatment for these rare types is similar to treatment for WM.

What can I do to get the best care?

Advocate for yourself. You have an important role to play in your care. In fact, you're more likely to get the care you want by asking questions and making shared decisions with your care team.

The NCCN Guidelines for Patients will help you understand cancer care. With better understanding, you'll be more prepared to discuss your care with your team and share your concerns. Many people feel more satisfied, confident, and less anxious when they play an active role in their care.

You may not know what to ask your care team. That's common. Each chapter in this book ends with an important section called Questions to ask. These suggested questions will help you get more information on all aspects of your care. Take the next step and keep reading to learn what is the best care for you.

2
Testing for WM

If your doctor suspects you have Waldenström macroglobulinemia (WM), you'll need several tests to confirm the diagnosis before you can begin treatment. Tests are also used to plan treatment, to find out how well treatment is working, and to check if cancer has come back after treatment.

This chapter describes what tests you may have and what you can expect during testing. You may have already had many of these tests. Some tests are used to diagnose WM. Others are used to see how well treatment is working. **See Guide 1.**

Symptoms and testing

A symptom is a problem or feeling that may signal an underlying disease or condition. Symptoms are different for everyone. No one gets all of the symptoms of WM. Some people don't get any symptoms. Even after diagnosis, some people may not have symptoms for years.

Although not everyone with WM has symptoms, many people are eventually diagnosed with WM because their symptoms motivate or lead them to be tested. For instance, two of the most common symptoms of WM are fatigue and weakness. **See Guide 2.**

But fatigue and weakness are also common symptoms of many other cancers and illnesses. So tests are necessary to identify whether these symptoms are caused by WM

Physical exam

One of the first tests you'll have is a physical. This is a hands-on examination. Your doctor may feel your neck for swollen lymph nodes (glands) or press your abdomen to find any enlarged organs, like your spleen or liver.

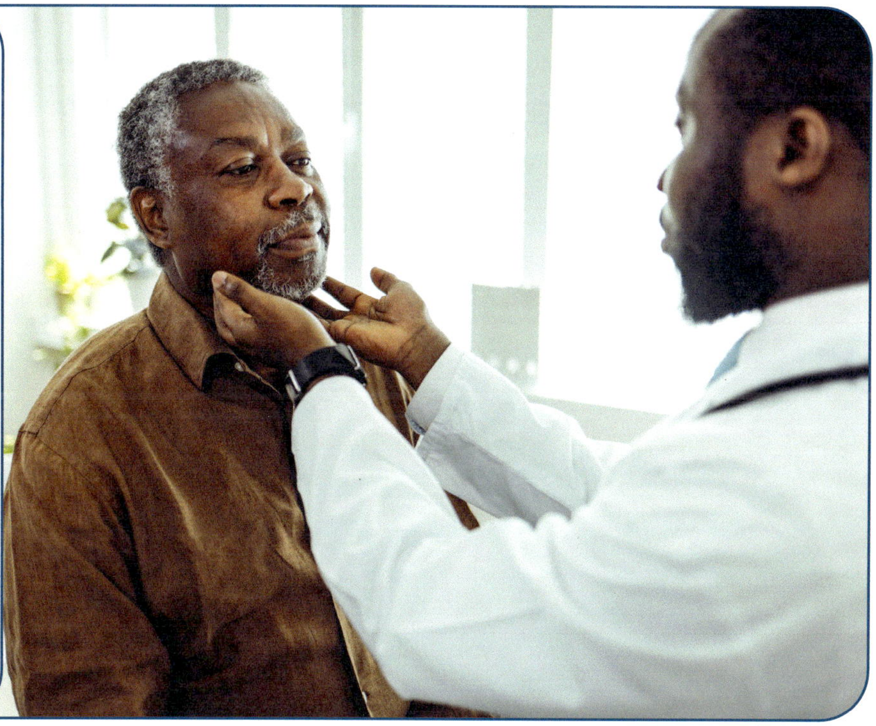

Guide 1
Tests for Waldenström macroglobulinemia

Necessary tests	Health history and physical exam
	Blood tests • Complete blood count • IgM and other immunoglobulins in blood • Liver and kidney function
	Bone marrow biopsy and lab tests • Bone marrow analysis (for WM cells) • Test to detect proteins (sIgM CD19, CD20, and others) on the surface of lymphoplasmacytic cells • Genetic test (for *MYD88* mutation)
	Imaging test(s) of the chest, abdomen, and pelvis • CT scan or FDG-PET/CT scan
Tests used in certain cases	Other blood tests • Blood viscosity • Cold agglutinins • Cryoglobulins
	Bone marrow biopsy and lab tests • Genetic test (for *CXCR4* mutation) • Bone marrow or fat biopsy (for amyloidosis)
	Virus tests • Hepatitis B • Hepatitis C • HIV
	Neurological tests • Electromyogram and nerve conduction study • Test for antibodies that affect the nervous system
	Eye exam
	Urine tests • 24-hour urine collection (for amyloidosis)

or by something else. In addition, symptoms can stem from a health condition related to WM. This is why tests are so important—they're used to find out what's underlying your symptoms. **See Guide 3.**

Now let's look at which tests you'll need to identify WM.

Blood tests

Blood tests play an important role in diagnosing and planning treatment for WM.

Blood tests are done in order to:

- **Count the number of cells in your blood,** including white blood cells, red blood cells, and platelets. This is called a complete blood count. Blood counts are often low in people with WM, which may indicate anemia. Anemia means your body doesn't have enough red blood cells to keep it working normally.
- **Measure the antibodies in your blood,** including the types and amounts of them. People with WM often have a high level of IgM antibodies and low levels of other antibodies (IgA and IgG). The IgM level can also be used during and after treatment to monitor how well your treatment is working. If the IgM antibodies in your blood are trending downward over time, your WM is likely getting better. If

Guide 2
Common symptoms of Waldenström macroglobulinemia

Fatigue	Easy bruising or bleeding
Weakness	Nosebleeds or bleeding gums
Fever	Headaches
Loss of appetite	Dizziness
Night sweats	Confusion
Unexpected weight loss	Infections
Numbness or painful tingling ("pins and needles") in hands and feet	Blurred vision or vision loss
Swollen lymph nodes	Swollen abdomen
Shortness of breath	Sensitivity to cold

Guide 3
WM complications and their symptoms

Complication	Description	Common symptoms
Amyloidosis	Buildup of abnormal protein (abnormal antibodies)	• Fatigue • Unexpected weight loss • Swelling of legs, ankles, or tongue • Numbness, tingling, or pain in hands or feet • Shortness of breath
Anemia	Low red blood cell count	• Fatigue • Dizziness • Racing heartbeat • Pale or yellow skin
Cold agglutinin disease	Destruction of red blood cells at lower body temperatures	• Fatigue • Shortness of breath • Racing heartbeat • Painful bluish fingers or toes • Yellowish skin and eyes • Dark urine
Cryoglobulinemia	Blockage of blood vessels during cold temperatures	• Purple or red skin lesions • Joint pain • Weakness • Change in color of hands or feet in cold temperatures • Numbness, tingling, or pain in hands or feet
Hyperviscosity syndrome	Thickening of the blood	• Nosebleeds or bleeding gums • Headache • Blurry vision • Blood clots • Dizziness • Vertigo • Chest pain • Shortness of breath
Peripheral neuropathy	Nerve damage caused by IgM antibodies	• Numbness, tingling, burning sensation, or pain in hands or feet • Muscle weakness • Loss of balance

IgM antibodies are on an upward trend, it may mean your treatment isn't working and WM is getting worse.

- **Assess the thickness of your blood.** Too many IgM antibodies in the blood can cause it to thicken, an uncommon but serious condition called hyperviscosity syndrome. Hyperviscosity limits blood flow, sometimes causing tiny blood vessels to burst. This can affect many parts of the body and lead to symptoms like nosebleeds, headaches, blurry vision, and even heart and lung conditions.
- **Look for antibodies that react to cold temperatures.** In rare cases, a person with WM has abnormal, cold-sensitive antibodies called cryoglobulins or cold agglutinins in their blood. When their body drops below its normal temperature, the cryoglobulins or cold agglutinins clump together and block blood flow. Over time, having cryoglobulins in your blood (a condition called cryoglobulinemia) can damage blood vessels, tissues, and organs (especially the kidneys).
- **Check for chemicals in your blood** that can indicate whether your liver, kidneys, or other organs are not working properly.
- **Screen for diseases and infections.** Some targeted therapies can wake up (reactivate) viruses like hepatitis B. If this happens, it can harm your liver. Hepatitis C infection is also linked to cryoglobulinemia. A blood test will show if you've had hepatitis in the past or if you have it now.

Bone marrow tests

If blood tests point to a high level of abnormal IgM, the next test should look for WM cells in bone marrow. Bone marrow is the sponge-like center of most bones where blood cells are made. Finding WM cells in the bone marrow indicates a diagnosis of WM.

To find out if your bone marrow contains these cells, a small amount of marrow needs to be removed from your body and tested. Bone marrow has both liquid and solid portions. So testing is done in two ways:

- **Bone marrow aspiration** removes a small amount of liquid bone marrow.
- **Bone marrow biopsy** removes a small amount of the solid portion of bone marrow.

These procedures are usually done at the same time in a hospital, clinic, or doctor's office. The marrow samples are removed from the back of the hip bone. You can usually go home the same day. You may have some bruising, tenderness, or pain in your lower back for a few days afterward.

After the biopsy, your bone marrow samples will be tested by a hematopathologist. A hematopathologist is an expert at diagnosing diseases of the blood and bone marrow.

The hematopathologist looks for at least 3 things:

Waldenström cells in your bone marrow

First, the hematopathologist will look at the cells of your bone marrow with a microscope. If you have Waldenström, your bone marrow may have a lot of WM cells (abnormal lymphocytes, plasma cells, and lymphoplasmacytic cells) as well as a shortage of healthy blood cells.

Proteins on the surface of lymphoplasmacytic cells

The bone marrow samples are also examined for specific proteins that are typically present—or notably absent—on the surface of lymphoplasmacytic cells.

In people with WM, proteins named sIgM, CD19, and CD20 are usually found on these cells. But CD5, CD10, and CD23 proteins are usually missing.

Gene mutations linked with WM

Genes are pieces of DNA that contain instructions for how our cells develop, grow, and function. Genes directly determine traits like your height and eye color. They also indirectly influence functions like how your body responds to infection.

Sometimes genes undergo abnormal changes called mutations. Most mutations won't affect your health at all. But some mutations are harmful and can increase the risk of developing certain illnesses like cancer.

A mutation can occur all on its own (spontaneously) or as a result of exposure to harmful things in the environment. Although certain genetic mutations can be inherited, the mutations linked to WM aren't passed down from parents to children.

Bone marrow aspiration and biopsy

To diagnose WM, samples of liquid and solid bone marrow must be tested in a laboratory. The samples are usually taken from the back of the hip bone. A diagnosis of Waldenström is likely if the samples contain a high number of WM cells—abnormal lymphocytes, plasma cells, and lymphoplasmacytic cells.

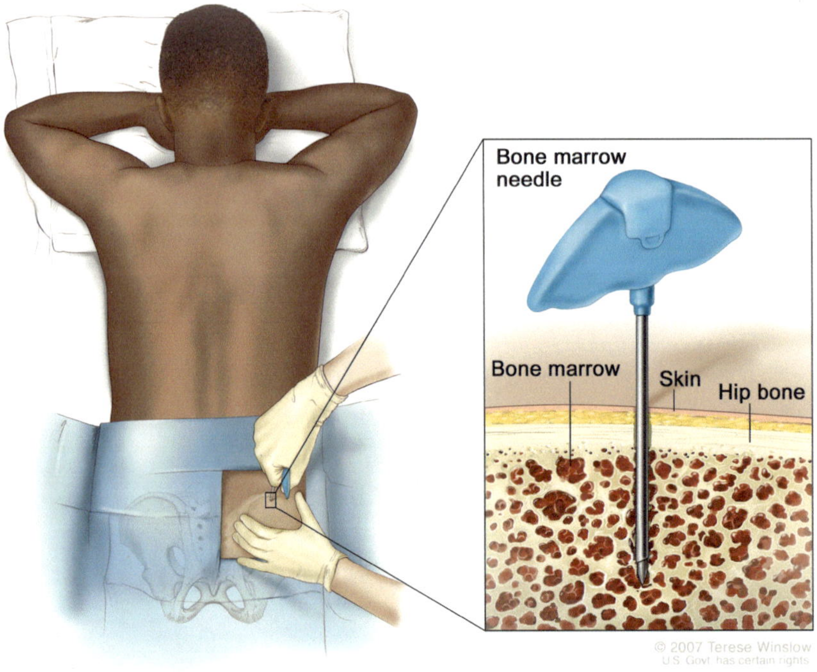

People with WM commonly have mutations in 2 genes:

- ***MYD88*** **–** Most people with WM have an abnormal (mutated) version of a gene called *MYD88*. Normally, the *MYD88* gene helps your immune system. But when *MYD88* is mutated, it helps cancer cells survive and multiply. Anyone who might have WM should be tested for this mutation.
- ***CXCR4*** **–** A mutation of the *CXCR4* gene occurs in about 4 out of 10 people who have WM. People with a *CXCR4* mutation may respond less well to treatment with a type of targeted therapy called Bruton's tyrosine kinase (BTK) inhibitors. If your care team is considering treatment with a BTK inhibitor such as ibrutinib, your bone marrow should be tested for *CXCR4* mutations.

Imaging tests

Imaging means taking detailed pictures (images) of the insides of the body. For WM, imaging scans can show if cancer has spread beyond the bone marrow. Imaging scans of your chest, abdomen, and pelvis help determine if your lymph nodes, spleen, or other organs are swollen with WM cells.

After diagnosis, imaging can also be used to track the progress of this cancer and how well your treatment is working.

CT scan

A widely used imaging test called a CT scan can provide information about the size, location, and extent of WM in the body. A CT scan takes many x-rays of the same body part from different angles. A computer combines all the x-ray pictures to make a cross-sectional image that's more detailed than a regular x-ray.

Computed tomography (CT)

CT scans can show if your lymph nodes or organs are enlarged. They're also helpful for determining if cancer has spread beyond the bone marrow.

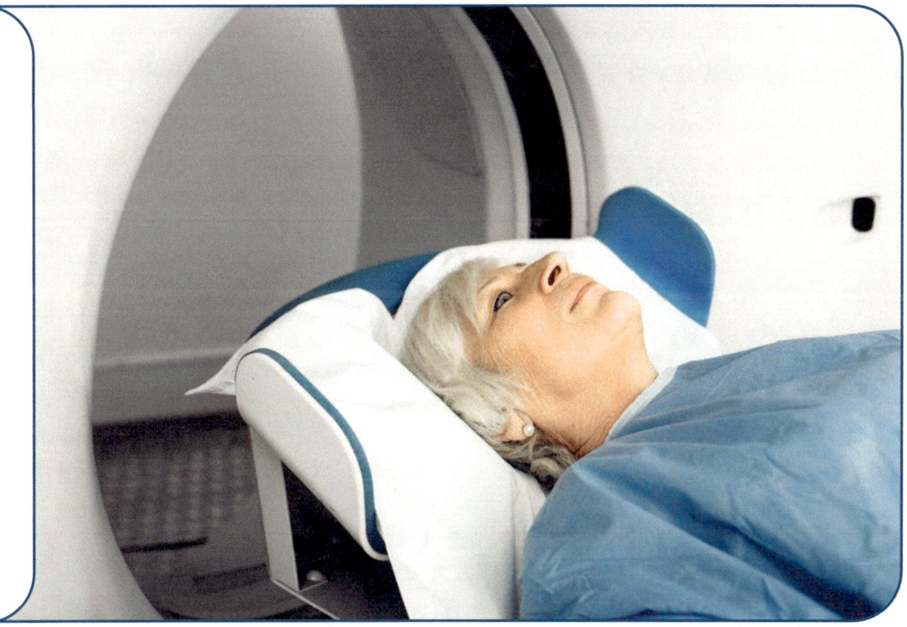

A substance called contrast is used to make parts of the body easier to see on a CT scan. The contrast is injected into your vein. Tell your care team if you've had an allergic reaction to contrast before.

PET/CT scan

Another imaging test called a PET scan highlights areas of the body where cells are more active than usual. And cancer cells are very active.

To create PET images, a substance called a tracer first needs to be injected into your body through a vein. The tracer makes cancer cells appear brighter in PET scans. The most commonly used tracer is called FDG.

A PET scan can show the extent of WM in your body. It can also show whether cancer cells are in areas like the bone marrow, lymph nodes, or organs.

CT and PET scans can be done separately or at the same time. When used together, it's called a PET/CT scan (or an FDG-PET/CT scan) and can provide even more information than either test used alone.

Other tests

In addition to blood tests, biopsies, and imaging, you may need other tests to learn more about your WM or its symptoms.

Urine tests

IgM can collect in urine as well as blood. Your doctor may order one or more tests of your urine to gain additional information. For example, a urine test may indicate a possible problem with your kidneys, which may not show up on a blood test.

Retinal exam

Hyperviscosity syndrome can cause eyesight problems such as blurred or double vision. If the level of IgM in your blood is high or if your doctor suspects hyperviscosity syndrome, you may have an exam of the back of your eye (retina) to check for any changes or bleeding.

Neurological tests

Your brain and spinal cord make up your central nervous system. The human body also has a peripheral nervous system, which includes all of the other nerves found throughout the body (peripheral nerves). These include nerves in muscles, glands, and organs.

Damage to the peripheral nerves can cause pain, numbness, tingling, burning sensation, or weakness. This is called peripheral neuropathy.

Peripheral neuropathy is common in people with WM and sometimes is the only source of symptoms. Damage often begins at the furthest points of the peripheral nervous system, the hands and feet. But it can also affect other parts of the body.

You may be referred to a neurologist if you have peripheral neuropathy. A neurologist is an expert in nervous system disorders. The neurologist may order tests that check your nerves and muscles to see how well they work together and whether there's any damage to them.

These may include:

- Nerve conduction study, which detects nerve damage by measuring how fast electrical impulses can travel through the nerves.
- Electromyography, which assesses the function of muscles and the nerves that control them.
- Testing for amyloidosis by using a special stain on a bone marrow sample or by removing and testing fat cells (a fat pad biopsy).
- Testing for antibodies of myelin-associated glycoprotein (MAG). MAG is an important protein needed to maintain a healthy nervous system.
- Testing for antibodies of ganglioside M1, a complex molecule in the nervous system.

You might also see a neurologist if you have symptoms related to a rare condition called Bing-Neel syndrome, in which lymphoplasmacytic cells enter the central nervous system (the brain and spinal cord).

Getting the diagnosis

Each test you have provides clues or pieces of the puzzle. Eventually, these clues lead to the diagnosis of the disease.

Waldenström macroglobulinemia can be diagnosed based on 2 key findings:

- Abnormal IgM in blood
- WM cells in bone marrow

Additional findings help support this diagnosis:

- Swollen lymph nodes or organs
- *MYD88* mutation

Where to get a diagnosis

Because Waldenström is so rare, even doctors who specialize in lymphoma may have seen few patients who have WM. If you can, go to a cancer specialist, cancer center, or hospital experienced in treating people with WM.

Electromyography

An electromyogram can detect nerve damage in people with symptoms of peripheral neuropathy, such as pain, tingling, burning sensation, or numbness.

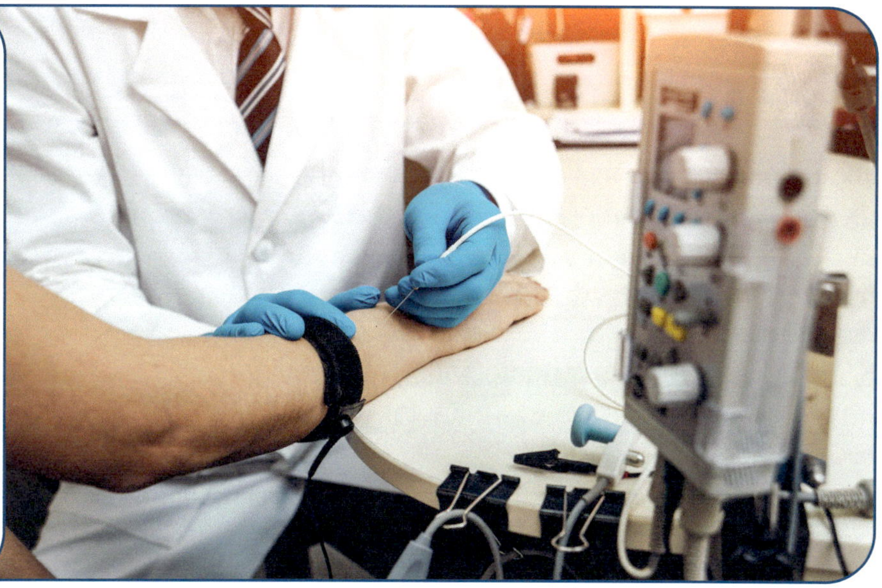

Resources are listed on page 40 that can help you find a WM specialist closest to you.

Notably, the International Waldenstrom's Macroglobulinemia Foundation maintains a list of physicians who are knowledgeable about WM. This directory can be found on the IWMF website (IWMF.com).

Do I need a second opinion?

WM is a slow-growing cancer, so there's usually time to have another cancer care provider review your test results and suggest a treatment plan. This is called getting a second opinion, and it's a normal part of cancer care. Even doctors get second opinions.

The IWMF directory is one place to look for a WM specialist who can provide a second opinion.

If you don't live near such a specialist, some cancer centers now provide virtual second opinions through their websites. For a list of NCCN affiliated cancer centers, turn to page 46 or see NCCN.org/member-institutions.

What's next?

Tests described in this chapter are used for diagnosis and planning treatment. To learn about what treatment you may need—or don't need—turn to the next chapter.

Keep in mind that *your* participation in making health care decisions is essential for you to receive the best treatment.

Key points

- Fatigue and weakness are 2 common symptoms of WM. Tests are necessary to identify whether they're caused by WM or by something else.
- Everyone with suspected WM should be tested for a mutated version of the *MYD88* gene.
- Too many IgM antibodies in the blood can cause it to thicken, a dangerous condition called hyperviscosity syndrome.
- Hyperviscosity of the blood can lead to symptoms like nosebleeds, headaches, vertigo, and blurry vision.
- Imaging scans can show if cancer has spread beyond the bone marrow to lymph nodes or other organs.
- The presence of abnormal IgM in blood and WM cells in bone marrow are the key findings to diagnose WM.

Questions to ask

- Where and when will my tests take place?
- How long will they take?
- How soon will I know the results and who will explain them to me?
- How often are these tests wrong?
- How do I get a second opinion?

3

Types of treatment for WM

Waldenström macroglobulinemia (WM) that's causing symptoms is treated with targeted therapy, chemotherapy, or both. But before these treatments, some people need excess immunoglobulin M (IgM) removed from their blood using a procedure called plasma exchange.

WM is different in every person. One person may have a lot of symptoms while another person has none.

If you have significant or bothersome symptoms related to WM, or your test results reveal a problem like hyperviscosity syndrome or a low blood cell count, then it's time to start treatment.

But if you don't have symptoms yet, you don't need treatment.

No symptoms, no treatment?

Once someone is diagnosed with cancer, they likely want to start treatment right away. But for WM, starting treatment may not be the best course of action.

It's important to remember that treatment won't get rid of Waldenström completely. Rather, treatment is for controlling the disease and relieving the symptoms caused by WM. So waiting until symptoms appear, or even until they become significant, is often the better strategy.

Why not start treatment anyway, just to be sure?

- Early treatment of WM won't prolong your life.
- Treatment can have side effects that lower your quality of life.
- Treatment may be inconvenient and have out-of-pocket costs.
- The longer you use a treatment, the more likely that WM will become resistant to it (able to overcome it).
- Better treatments may be available in the future.

You may not need to start treatment for months or years after diagnosis. Some people never need treatment.

Even people with manageable symptoms may prefer to delay treatment. That's because WM grows slowly and gradually. So you and your treatment team will have enough time to decide when treatment should begin. This is called "watchful waiting."

Watchful waiting

Some people call this "watch and worry," but their worry usually subsides after they get used to the routine.

Watchful waiting, also called active monitoring or observation, doesn't involve treatment. But you'll have regular checkups to make sure nothing has changed.

At each visit, you'll have tests to check the amount of IgM in your blood. A normal range is approximately 150 to 300 milligrams of IgM per deciliter of blood (mg/dL). How often you'll need to come in will be based on your symptoms and lab results. Some people will only need a checkup once or twice a year. Others will need visits every 3 months.

You may never develop symptoms in your lifetime. But if you do, be sure to tell your care team about them so you can get the proper treatment.

Primary treatment for Waldenström may begin when your symptoms become bothersome or they interfere with your daily life.

People who need immediate relief from symptoms, such as those with hyperviscosity syndrome, can have a procedure to reduce their IgM antibodies before starting primary therapy. This procedure is called a plasma exchange.

Who's on your care team?

Treating WM takes a team approach. Some members of your care team will be with you throughout your treatment, while others will be there for parts of it. Your team should communicate and work together to bring the best knowledge from each specialty.

Your team will be led by a hematologist-oncologist—an expert in treating blood cancers.

Other common team members include medical oncologists, neurologists, hematopathologists, ophthalmologists, nurses, pharmacists, physician assistants, patient navigators, social workers, and other specialists.

Plasma exchange

Plasma exchange doesn't treat Waldenström directly. Rather, it's a way to relieve the symptoms of WM. It also helps your body prepare for primary therapy, such as targeted therapy or chemotherapy.

Plasma exchange involves a process called plasmapheresis that separates plasma from blood. Plasma is the liquid part of blood without the blood cells. Plasma contains the serum, a clear, yellowish liquid that carries nutrients, waste products, and proteins like immunoglobulins. In people with WM, plasma contains abnormal IgM.

In a plasma exchange, your "old" plasma—high in IgM—is removed and then replaced with "new" plasma that contains no IgM. With no extra IgM in your body, your symptoms will improve quickly.

Who should have plasma exchange?

- People with symptoms of hyperviscosity syndrome should have plasma exchange as soon as possible. After plasma exchange, therapy should be started right away.

- People with a very high level of IgM (6,000 mg/dL or higher), even if they don't have symptoms of hyperviscosity, should be considered for plasma exchange.
- People with a high level of IgM (4,000 mg/dL or higher) who will be treated with rituximab (Rituxan) can have plasma exchange to prevent a dangerous increase in IgM after rituximab treatment.

Notably, treatment with rituximab can cause IgM to increase suddenly (IgM "flare"). This sharp spike in IgM can lead to hyperviscosity syndrome and worsening of other complications. So lowering the level of IgM before taking rituximab reduces the risk of potential symptoms.

What happens during a plasma exchange?

A plasma exchange can take 2 to 3 hours. You'll sit in a reclining chair or lie on a bed. During this process:

1. An intravenous (IV) line is put into a vein in your arm or in your chest (central catheter) to remove some of your blood.
2. The blood goes into a machine that removes the plasma from your blood a little at a time.
3. Plasma from a donor or a liquid substitute is mixed with the removed blood and returned to you through the IV.

What happens after a plasma exchange?

After plasma exchange, the level of IgM in your blood will be monitored closely. You'll continue to have plasma exchange sessions (typically 2 or 3 within days of each other) until your IgM level drops significantly and your hyperviscosity symptoms go away. These effects are short-lived, though, so your primary therapy should begin soon after plasma exchange ends.

Plasma exchange

Plasma exchange removes IgM from your blood. In this process, blood is drawn from your body into a machine that separates the plasma (which carries IgM) from the blood cells. New plasma (with no IgM) is combined with your removed blood cells and returned to your body.

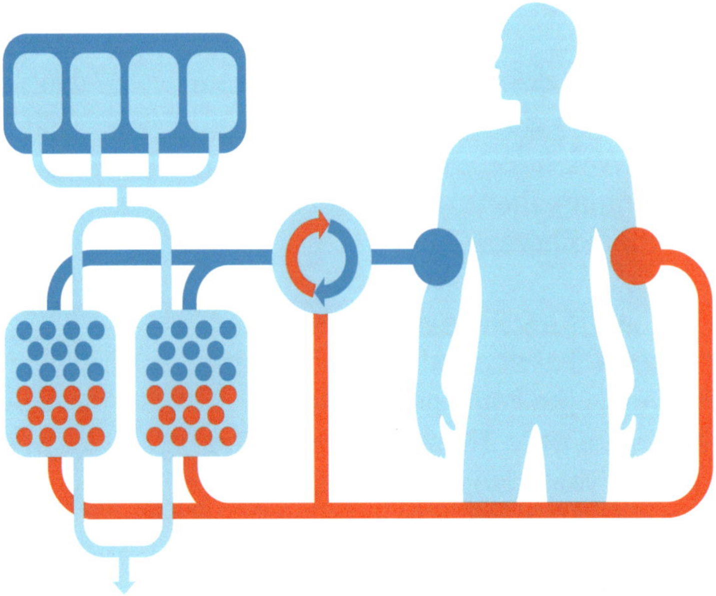

If symptoms of hyperviscosity return, you can have plasma exchange again. It's common to have plasma exchange more than once before primary therapy.

Primary therapy

Primary therapy is the first treatment you receive. The goals of primary therapy are to relieve your symptoms and reduce the risk of damage to your organs.

The two main types of primary therapy used to treat WM are targeted therapy and chemotherapy.

- Targeted therapy finds and attacks specific types of cancer cells.
- Chemotherapy stops the growth of cancer cells, either by killing the cells or stopping them from dividing.

These two types of therapy may be used individually or combined with one another.

There are 4 drug or drug combinations that are preferred for primary therapy. Preferred treatments have the most evidence they work better and may be safer than other therapies. **See Guide 4.**

Although preferred treatments are often chosen first, other recommended treatments can also be a good choice. **See Guide 5.** Other recommended treatments may not work quite as well as preferred therapies for some people, but overall they're still useful for treating WM.

Guide 4 **Preferred primary treatments for WM** *(in alphabetical order)*
Bendamustine and rituximab
Ibrutinib
Ibrutinib and rituximab
Zanubrutinib

Guide 5 **Other recommended primary treatments for WM** *(in alphabetical order)*
Bendamustine
Bortezomib, rituximab, and dexamethasone
Carfilzomib, rituximab, and dexamethasone
Ixazomib, rituximab, and dexamethasone
Rituximab
Rituximab, cyclophosphamide, and dexamethasone
Rituximab, cyclophosphamide, bortezomib, and dexamethasone
Rituximab, cyclophosphamide, and prednisone

Let's look at each type of treatment used for primary therapy:

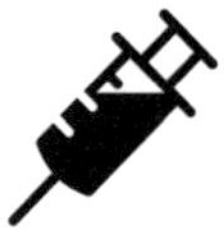

Rituximab

Rituximab (Rituxan) is a monoclonal antibody therapy—a targeted therapy that uses a single type of antibody to find and bind to cancer cells.

How it works

Your body makes natural antibodies to fight harmful invaders like bacteria, viruses, and even cancer cells.

Rituximab is an antibody made in a lab. It targets a protein called CD20. This protein is commonly found on the surface of cancerous blood cells (including WM cells) and on some normal blood cells. Once rituximab finds CD20, it attaches itself to it. Then rituximab acts like a beacon to help your immune system find and attack those cells.

Rituximab also targets CD20 protein on some healthy blood cells, which results in a number of the drug's side effects.

How it's given

Rituximab is a liquid that is slowly injected into a vein or sometimes injected just under the skin. Your treatment team will figure out the dose (amount given), how long it will be given, and how often you'll receive it.

Rituximab is often given in combination with other therapies. You may also receive medication beforehand to prevent a common response called an infusion reaction.

Infusion reaction

Infusion means the medicine is put directly into the bloodstream. An infusion reaction is when the immune system has a bad or overreactive response to an infusion. Infusion reactions are common when receiving rituximab, often when receiving it for the first time.

The reaction can happen during the infusion itself or the day afterward. It can come on like a sudden allergy attack, and may cause itchy skin, rash, hives, cough, chills, fever, scratchy or tight throat, swollen lips or tongue, or shortness of breath.

Severe infusion reactions are less common but more dangerous. A severe reaction can cause anaphylaxis, low blood pressure, irregular heartbeat, heart attack, or even death.

To prevent or reduce an infusion reaction, you'll receive anti-allergy medicine and acetaminophen (Tylenol), and maybe a steroid. Also, the infusion itself may be slowed down so your body can absorb the medicine more gradually.

Often, infusion reactions aren't as bad the second time receiving rituximab. But if you continue to have bad reactions, you can switch to a different treatment.

IgM flare

Rituximab can cause the level of IgM in your blood to increase significantly and remain high for months. This is called an IgM flare. The increase in IgM can worsen other side effects and cause blood to thicken (hyperviscosity syndrome). If blood thickens enough, serious symptoms may develop, such as abnormal bleeding, blurry vision, headaches or dizziness.

If the level of IgM in your blood is high (above 4,000 mg/dL) or you have hyperviscosity symptoms before starting treatment with rituximab, your team may recommend having a plasma exchange first. This is done to help prevent hyperviscosity symptoms from starting or getting worse.

If your IgM level increases significantly after starting treatment with rituximab, you might have another plasma exchange, even if you don't have symptoms.

Other side effects of rituximab

High blood pressure, nausea, chest (respiratory) infections, weakness, body aches, joint pain, fever, and chills.

BTK inhibitors

BTK inhibitors are another kind of targeted therapy. BTK inhibitors commonly used for treating Waldenström include:

- Acalabrutinib (Calquence)
- Ibrutinib (Imbruvica)
- Zanubrutinib (Brukinsa)

How they work

WM starts in immune cells (lymphocytes) called B cells. B cells contain a protein called Bruton's tyrosine kinase (BTK). The BTK protein sends signals that help B cells multiply and stay alive. But even when B cells become cancerous, BTK continues to help these cells to thrive. So they're able to create even more cancerous B cells.

"Be your own advocate. Ask a lot of questions, even the ones you're afraid to ask. You have to ensure you make the best decisions for your particular situation."

BTK inhibitors are drugs that block (inhibit) BTK from working, which helps stop cancer cells from surviving and multiplying.

How they're given

BTK inhibitors are taken by mouth as a pill. Unlike chemotherapy, which is given periodically, BTK inhibitors are taken every day for long as they're effective for you.

Side effects of BTK inhibitors

BTK inhibitors can cause serious side effects. These include heart rhythm problems, high blood pressure, excessive bleeding, and chest infections (such as pneumonia).

Other common side effects of BTK inhibitors are nausea, diarrhea, fatigue, joint and muscle pain, headache, and skin rash.

Stopping BTK inhibitors suddenly can cause WM to return and to get worse quickly. Someone with WM who's planning to switch to a new treatment should continue taking their BTK inhibitor up until they start the next therapy. However, if you need to pause your BTK inhibitor due to a procedure or surgery, your doctor can tell you how to do it safely.

In people who have a *CXCR4* mutation, the BTK inhibitor ibrutinib may not work very well. Your bone marrow or blood should be tested for *CXCR4* mutations if your team is planning treatment with ibrutinib.

Proteasome inhibitors

Proteasome inhibitors are a type of targeted therapy that shuts down cellular activity, particularly the activity in cancer cells. Three proteasome inhibitors are available for the treatment of WM:

- Bortezomib (Velcade)
- Carfilzomib (Kyprolis)
- Ixazomib (Ninlaro)

How they work

All cells in the body contain tiny "machines" called proteasomes. Proteasomes have been nicknamed the cell's garbage disposal because they grind up, recycle, and get rid of a cell's waste.

Drugs called proteasome inhibitors stop proteasomes from "taking out the trash." With proteasomes shut down, the waste gradually piles up inside the cancer cell. When the cell can't hold any more, it bursts and dies.

How they're given

Bortezomib and carfilzomib are liquid medicines given as injections. Bortezomib is injected preferably just under the skin once a week. Carfilzomib is slowly injected into a vein once (or twice) a week. Ixazomib is a capsule taken by mouth usually once a week. Proteasome inhibitors are given in combination with rituximab and dexamethasone.

How targeted therapy works: One example

Targeted therapy drugs work in different ways. One way is by blocking a process that keeps the WM cell alive. One such process: Proteasomes that clear out waste proteins in WM cells.

But a targeted drug can block proteasomes from carrying out this process. If the proteasomes are halted, then the waste proteins build up inside the cells.

Eventually, the WM cells become overloaded with waste proteins and are destroyed.

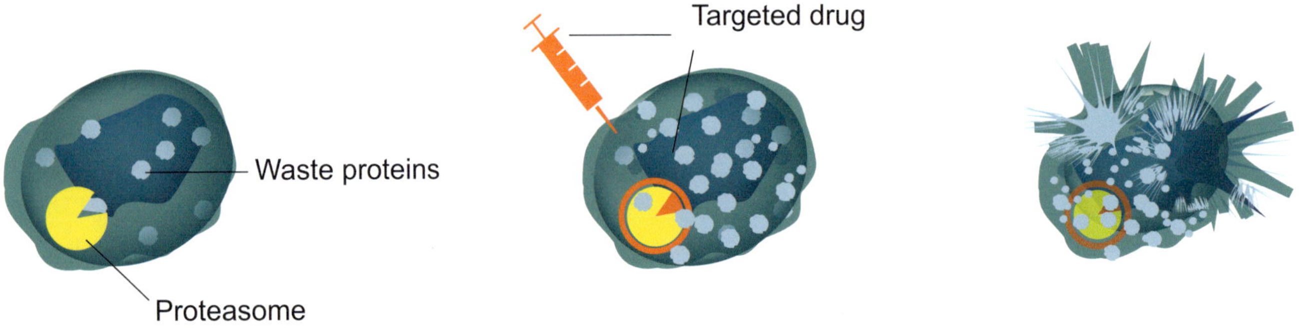

You'll continue to receive these treatments for as long as directed by your provider.

Shingles

Shingles is a potential side effect of proteasome inhibitors. Shingles is a painful skin rash caused by the same virus that causes chickenpox. Proteasome inhibitors can reactivate this virus. Shingles often appears as blisters on one side of the body or face. Shingles may be more common in people with weakened immune systems.

If a proteasome inhibitor is part of your treatment plan, your provider may recommend you get the shingles vaccine. Another precaution—you should take an antiviral medication during proteasome treatment and for a few months after (whether you got the vaccine or not) to reduce the risk of shingles.

Other side effects of proteasome inhibitors

Bortezomib may cause peripheral neuropathy in some people. In people who already have neuropathy, bortezomib can make it worse. Other common side effects include diarrhea, nausea, vomiting, constipation, and reduced appetite.

Carfilzomib may cause serious damage to the heart, lungs and kidneys, especially in older adults. If you're taking this medication, immediately report any symptoms coming from the heart, lungs, or kidneys.

Side effects of treatment

Therapy for WM can kill cancer cells, but may also destroy normal cells. Damage to normal cells causes potentially harsh side effects.

Side effects are different for everyone. Some people have many side effects while others have few. The risk for side effects often depends on the specific medicine given, the dose, and the length of treatment.

Most side effects appear when treatment starts and then stop when it's over. However, some side effects may continue after treatment or may appear years after your treatment is over.

Tell your treatment team if you have any new or worsening symptoms. There are ways to help you feel better. There are also ways to prevent some side effects.

Chemotherapy

Chemotherapy treats cancer by killing fast-dividing cells throughout the body. Cancer cells divide rapidly, but so do some normal cells. Damage to normal cells can cause potentially harsh side effects.

How it's given

Chemotherapy is often given in cycles over several months. One cycle includes several treatment days followed by a longer period of rest. This rest period allows your body to recover before you start the next cycle. Each cycle usually lasts for a few weeks.

The chemotherapy medicines used to treat WM are given as IV infusions. This means they are slowly put into your bloodstream through a vein.

Two types of chemotherapy are used for WM:

- Alkylating agents – Bendamustine (Treanda and Bendeka) and cyclophosphamide (Cytoxan) belong to a group of chemotherapy drugs called alkylating agents. Alkylating agents damage cell DNA to prevent the cells from copying themselves.
- Antimetabolites – Cladribine and fludarabine belong to a group of chemotherapy medicines called antimetabolites. Antimetabolites work by switching places with the building blocks of the cell's DNA, sabotaging its ability to divide and multiply.

Cladribine and fludarabine can be very damaging to the rapidly-dividing stem cells in bone marrow. So if there is even a small chance that you may have a procedure called a stem cell rescue in the future, your doctor should avoid or limit the use of cladribine and fludarabine.

Stem cell rescue is discussed in detail in *Chapter 4 – Therapies for previously treated WM*.

Side effects of chemotherapy

Some of the common side effects of these chemotherapy medicines are fever, chills, fatigue, nausea, vomiting, diarrhea, headache, loss of appetite, cough, lower back or side pain, increased risk of infection, and unusual bleeding or bruising.

Steroids

Steroids (short for corticosteroids) are used widely in medicine to reduce swelling and inflammation. They also have a number of uses for treating WM:

- Steroids increase the effectiveness of chemotherapy when these drugs are used together.
- Steroids are poisonous to B cells (the immune cells where WM begins).
- Steroids help reduce side effects of chemotherapy, such as nausea and vomiting.
- Steroids can lower the body's immune response, which may help prevent an allergic reaction to rituximab.

The steroids used for WM treatment are dexamethasone and prednisone. They may be given as a pill, a liquid, or an IV injection.

Side effects of steroids

Common side effects of steroids are feeling hungry, trouble sleeping, slow wound healing, upset stomach, muscle weakness, and weight gain. Steroids can also cause high blood sugar levels (hyperglycemia). Steroids make some people feel irritable and cranky. Changes in mood can happen from day to day.

Other care before and during therapy

IgA and IgG monitoring

Treatment with many of the recommended systemic therapy regimens can cause the levels of two antibodies (IgA and IgG) to become too low. You'll have blood tests during treatment to make sure these antibodies aren't depleted.

However, if you develop symptoms related to low IgG, such as repeated infections, then you can receive an infusion of additional healthy IgG antibodies.

Pneumocystis pneumonia prevention

Pneumocystis pneumonia is a fungal infection of the lungs. It occurs most often in people with weak immune systems. Your doctor may prescribe a medication to lower the risk of pneumocystis pneumonia before you begin treatment with certain drug combinations.

Clinical trials

Joining a clinical trial is also an option for treating WM. Participating in a clinical trial allows you to get treatment while also helping cancer researchers learn more about this rare disease.

A clinical trial is a type of medical research study. After being developed and tested in a lab, potential new ways of fighting cancer need to be studied in people.

If found to be safe and effective in a clinical trial, a drug, device, or treatment approach may be approved by the U.S. Food and Drug Administration (FDA).

Everyone with cancer should carefully consider all of the treatment options available for their cancer type, including standard treatments and clinical trials. Talk to your doctor about whether a clinical trial may make sense for you.

Phases

Most cancer clinical trials focus on treatment and are done in phases.

- **Phase 1** trials study the safety and side effects of an investigational drug or treatment approach.
- **Phase 2** trials study how well the drug or approach works against a specific type of cancer.
- **Phase 3** trials test the drug or approach against a standard treatment. If the results are good, it may be approved by the FDA.
- **Phase 4** trials study the safety and benefit of an FDA-approved treatment.

Who can enroll?

It depends on the clinical trial's rules, called eligibility criteria. The rules may be about age, cancer type and stage, treatment history, or general health. They ensure that participants are alike in specific ways and that the trial is as safe as possible for the participants.

Informed consent

Clinical trials are managed by a research team. This group of experts will review the study with you in detail, including its purpose and the risks and benefits of joining.

All of this information is also provided in an informed consent form. Read the form carefully and ask questions before signing it. Take time to discuss it with people you trust. Keep in mind that you can leave and seek treatment outside of the clinical trial at any time.

Will I get a placebo?

Placebos (inactive versions of real medicines) are almost never used alone in cancer clinical trials. It's common to receive either a placebo with a standard treatment, or a new drug with a standard treatment. You'll be informed, verbally and in writing, if a placebo is part of a clinical trial before you enroll.

Are clinical trials free?

There is no fee to enroll in a clinical trial. The study sponsor pays for costs related to the research. But you'll still be asked to cover typical or standard-of-care medical costs. This care is often billed to your insurance. You'll also need to pay for any other services, like transportation or childcare, due to extra appointments.

Finding a clinical trial

In the United States

NCCN Cancer Centers
NCCN.org/cancercenters

The National Cancer Institute (NCI)
cancer.gov/about-cancer/treatment/clinical-trials/search

Worldwide

The U.S. National Library of Medicine (NLM)
clinicaltrials.gov/

Need help finding a clinical trial?

NCI's Cancer Information Service (CIS)
1.800.4.CANCER (1.800.422.6237)
cancer.gov/contact

Testing after treatment

After primary therapy, you'll have tests to check how well the treatment worked. Testing will likely include a physical exam, blood tests, and imaging scans of your chest, abdomen, and pelvis. You'll also be asked whether you have any new or worsening symptoms.

IgM level suggests treatment effect

The level of IgM in your blood is the main indicator of how well your treatment worked. A lower IgM level typically means your treatment is working. You may need 2 (or more) separate blood tests to confirm your IgM level.

However, IgM level doesn't always reflect the amount of cancer cells destroyed. Some medicines can cause IgM levels to fluctuate, making it difficult to know how much the treatment reduced the cancer.

For example, rituximab (Rituxan) can cause IgM levels to go up for weeks or months (IgM flare). Bortezomib (Velcade) can cause IgM levels to go down without killing cancer cells, giving a false impression that treatment was effective. And some medicines can simply take longer than others to lower IgM levels.

Biopsy if IgM is unclear

Sometimes there can be a mismatch between the level of IgM in your blood and how well treatment is working. If your symptoms are getting better and you seem to be responding to treatment, but the level of IgM in your blood is still high, your provider may order a bone marrow biopsy to get a clearer picture of how much cancer you have left. (See *Transformation* sidebar.)

That's why IgM level isn't the only factor used to determine if treatment was successful.

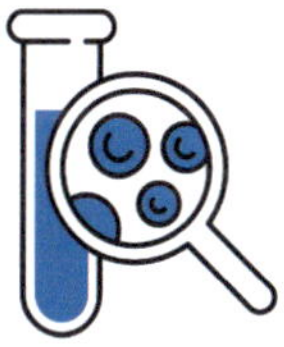

Transformation

While uncommon, it's possible for a slow-growing lymphoma like WM to transform into a fast-growing lymphoma. One reason your care team may want to do a biopsy is to rule out transformation into a fast-growing lymphoma.

A change in your symptoms may be a sign of transformation. Symptoms include unexplained fever, night sweats, or significant weight loss. Other symptoms are enlarged lymph nodes and organs.

If testing finds that WM has transformed, read about Diffuse Large B-Cell Lymphomas at NCCN.org/patientguidelines and on the NCCN Patient Guides for Cancer app.

When does treatment stop?

Whether you're finished with treatment depends on the type of treatment chosen and how well it worked.

If your IgM drops to a normal level and you have no symptoms, your treatment worked well.

If someone's IgM continues to rise and their symptoms remain or get worse, their treatment didn't work at all. This response is called progressive disease because the cancer is still advancing (progressing).

For many people with WM, their response to treatment ranges somewhere in between these two extremes. Whatever the case may be, further treatment depends on whether or not you have symptoms after primary therapy:

You have symptoms after therapy

If your symptoms remain or get worse after primary therapy, then you'll continue to have treatment. Typically, your doctor will ask you to switch to a different treatment than the one you had for primary therapy. The silver lining is that there are a lot of other treatments available. (Read more about this in *Chapter 4: Therapies for previously treated WM.*)

You don't have symptoms after therapy

If your symptoms of WM go away, then you won't need further treatment right now.

(Symptoms from another, unrelated disease—diabetes, for example—may not go away.) However, if you've been taking a BTK inhibitor, you'll need to keep taking it indefinitely unless symptoms return.

Your doctor or care team will continue to check your IgM level periodically throughout the rest of your life. These visits will be more frequent at first (every few months for several years). Besides these visits, you'll be able to live your life much like you did before you were diagnosed with WM.

If your IgM level starts to increase again, it doesn't mean you automatically need more treatment. More treatment is only needed if symptoms return. (Read more about this in *Chapter 4: Therapies for previously treated WM.*)

What's next?

WM is a lifelong disease. It's common for symptoms of WM to eventually return (relapse) after therapy and require further treatment.

People with WM whose therapy didn't work also require more treatment. The next chapter explains what therapies are available when symptoms of WM come back or haven't gone away.

Key points

- WM only requires treatment if it's causing symptoms.
- Watchful waiting involves regular checkups, not treatment.
- People with symptoms of hyperviscosity syndrome should have plasma exchange right away to provide relief and prevent organ damage.
- People without symptoms of hyperviscosity but with a high IgM level might also have plasma exchange before starting treatment that includes rituximab.
- Targeted therapy, chemotherapy, or both are used to treat WM that is causing symptoms.
- If your symptoms remain or get worse after primary therapy, you can have more treatment—but usually a different treatment than what you already had.

Questions to ask

- How soon should I start treatment? How long does treatment take?
- How much time do I have to think about my options or to get a second opinion?
- Do my age, general health, or other factors affect my treatment options?
- What risks or side effects are there to the treatments you suggest? What can I do to reduce side effects?
- How much experience do you have treating WM?

4

Therapies for previously treated WM

Waldenström macroglobulinemia (WM) often returns at some point after treatment. This is called a relapse. Relapsed WM is treated with therapy you've had before or with a different therapy altogether.

Waldenström macroglobulinemia often comes back eventually—perhaps many months or even many years after prior treatment. This is called a relapse, and it requires treatment of its own. For some people, WM relapses more than once.

In other people, Waldenström can become resistant to treatment, or the effects of treatment don't last very long. These people can request a different treatment.

People whose symptoms haven't gone away, or whose WM continues to progress after primary treatment, need further treatment as well.

Options for further treatment

Although you've had treatment already, you still have many other treatments to choose from.

The choice of treatment may depend on which treatment you had before, whether it worked or how long it worked, and what side effects it caused.

Your personal preferences about treatment should also be considered. Ask your team about how different drugs are administered, how long treatment lasts, what side effects are possible, whether it's covered by your insurance, and any other concerns you have.

Same treatment

You may be offered the same treatment you had for primary therapy, especially if the treatment was effective for a long time and it didn't cause significant side effects.

Some chemotherapy medicines should be chosen carefully when given more than once. The more you use them, the more toxic they become to your body.

Different treatment

Rather than repeating primary therapy, a different type of treatment is recommended if:

- WM relapses within 2 years after primary treatment
- Symptoms of WM don't go away after primary treatment
- WM gets worse (progresses) after primary treatment
- Your primary therapy was very harsh or caused severe side effects

The preferred therapies for previously treated WM are listed in **Guide 6.** Other recommended therapies are listed in **Guide 7.**

Although not listed here, additional treatments are also available for use in certain circumstances.

Guide 6 **Preferred therapies for previously treated WM** *(in alphabetical order)*
Bendamustine and rituximab
Ibrutinib
Ibrutinib and rituximab
Rituximab, cyclophosphamide, and dexamethasone
Zanubrutinib

Guide 7 **Other recommended therapies for previously treated WM** *(in alphabetical order)*
Acalabrutinib
Bortezomib, rituximab, and dexamethasone
Ixazomib, rituximab, and dexamethasone
Rituximab, cyclophosphamide, and prednisone
Venetoclax

If WM returns more than once, you may be offered a procedure called high-dose chemotherapy with autologous stem cell rescue (HDT/ASCR).

HDT/ASCR

High-dose chemotherapy (HDT) with autologous stem cell rescue (ASCR) is a treatment option only for certain people with relapsed WM. It's mainly used for people whose previous treatments didn't reduce their cancer (or didn't reduce it for very long) and for those who have WM with amyloidosis.

HDT/ASCR is an intense and complicated treatment. However, the concept is fairly simple: It destroys cancer cells in your body and replaces them with your own healthy cells.

The healthy cells involved are stem cells. A stem cell is a basic, immature cell that develops into other types of cells. The stem cells in HDT/ASCR are called hematopoietic (blood-forming) stem cells because they grow into mature blood cells.

Here's how HDT/ASCR works:

- **Preparation**: First, you're given injections of growth factors to boost your body's production of stem cells.
- **Collection**: Blood is removed from a vein in your arm into a medical device. The device separates (harvests) stem cells from your blood and returns the remaining blood to your other arm. The harvested stem cells are frozen and stored to keep them alive.
- **Destruction**: Next, you're given high doses of chemotherapy to destroy the cancer cells in your body. This also wipes out your immune system. Special precautions are taken to protect you from infection.

- **Transplantation**: After chemotherapy, your harvested stem cells are slowly returned through a vein to your bloodstream (transfusion). The transplanted stem cells travel to your bone marrow and gradually begin to grow new, healthy blood cells. (The transplanted cells "rescue" your bone marrow.)

HDT/ASCR is a demanding treatment. It also comes with the risk of chemotherapy side effects. It's not meant for everyone. Your treatment team will consider your overall health, your age, and other factors to decide if this procedure is right for you.

It's also important to know that certain chemotherapy medicines (fludarabine and cladribine) can damage stem cells. If your doctor thinks you're likely to have HDT/ASCR in the future, you should not have these medications as initial therapy.

Additional support

The main concern for most patients is to find a treatment that works. Having cancer is about more than just treatment, though. Cancer care can be a rollercoaster that includes many additional physical and emotional challenges. It's important to know that you can get support for these challenges.

High-dose chemotherapy with autologous stem cell rescue

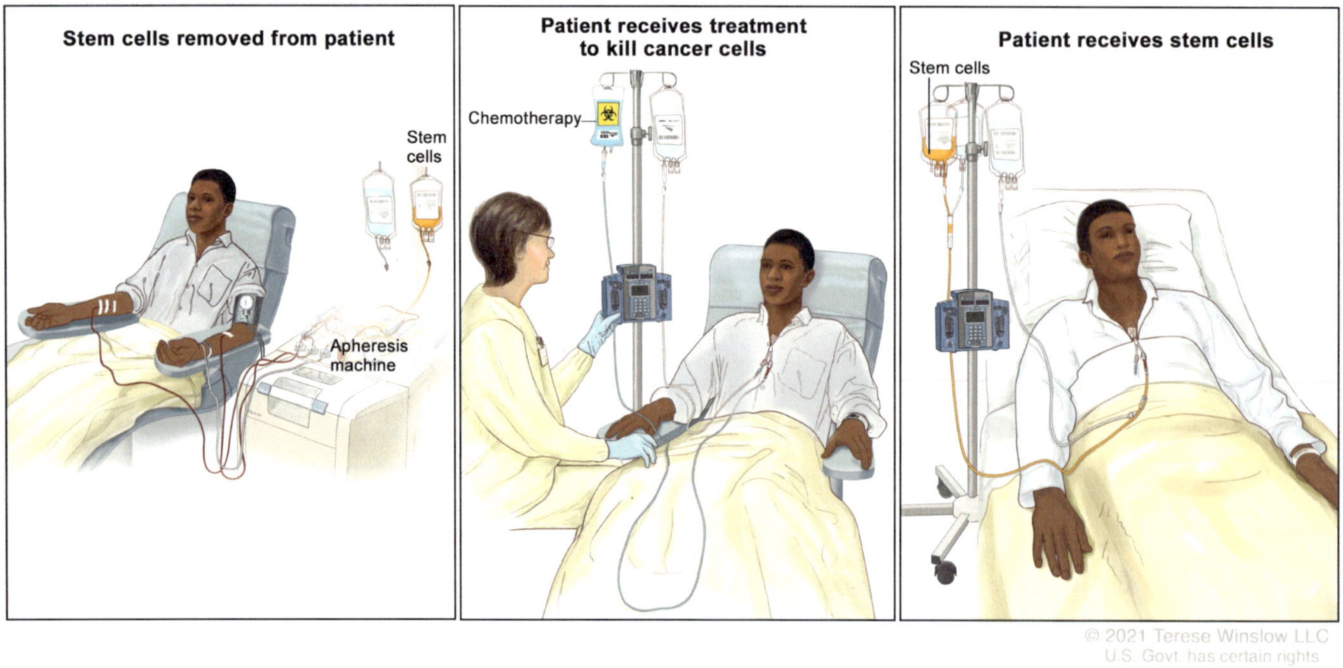

Survivorship

Survivorship focuses on the health and well-being of a person with cancer from diagnosis until the end of life. This includes the physical, mental, emotional, social, and financial effects of cancer that begin at diagnosis, continue through treatment and recovery, and arise afterward.

Survivorship also includes concerns about follow-up care, late effects of treatment, cancer recurrence, age-appropriate preventive care, and quality of life. Support from family members, friends, and caregivers is also an important part of survivorship.

Read more about survivorship at NCCN.org/patientguidelines and on the NCCN Patient Guides for Cancer app.

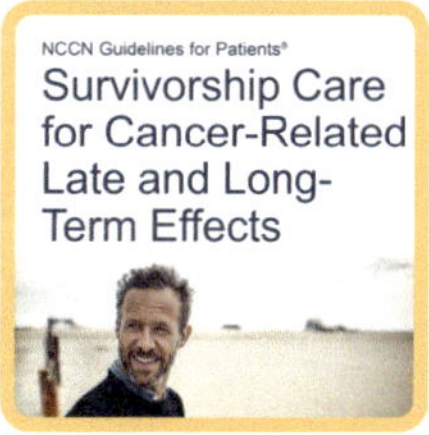

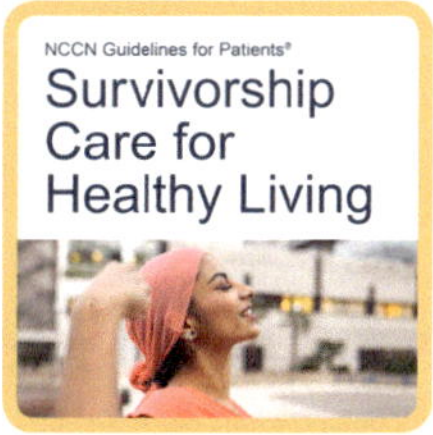

Supportive care

Supportive care helps improve your quality of life during and after cancer treatment. The goal of supportive care is to prevent or manage side effects and symptoms, like pain and cancer-related fatigue. Supportive care also addresses the mental, social, and spiritual concerns faced by those with cancer.

Supportive care is given at any stage of disease, not just at the end of life. It's available to everyone with cancer and their families. Palliative care is another name for supportive care.

Supportive care can also help with:

- Making treatment decisions
- Coordinating your care
- Paying for care
- Planning for advanced care and end of life

Ask questions and reach out to your treatment team if you need more information about supportive care. Some medical centers have patient navigators or other staff members who coordinate nonclinical supportive care.

More information on supportive care is available at NCCN.org/patientguidelines and on the NCCN Patient Guides for Cancer app.

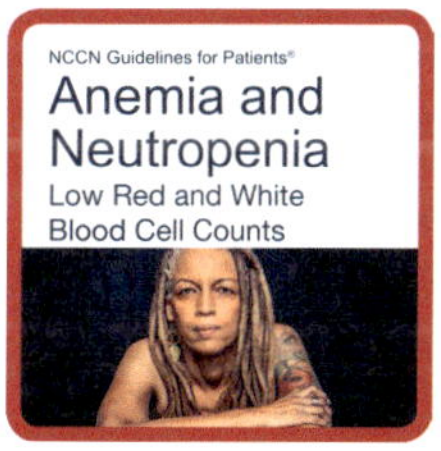

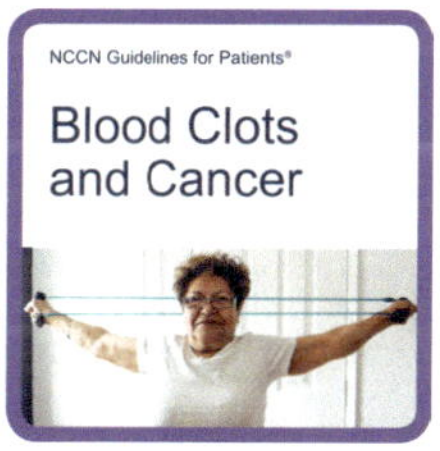

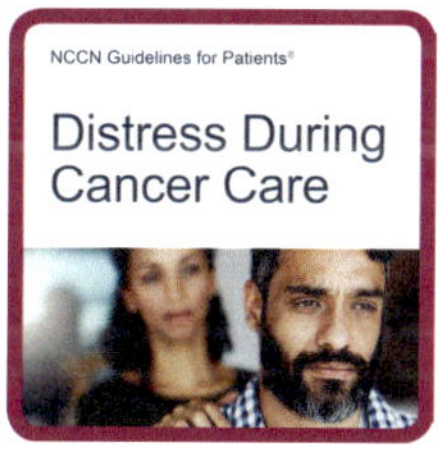

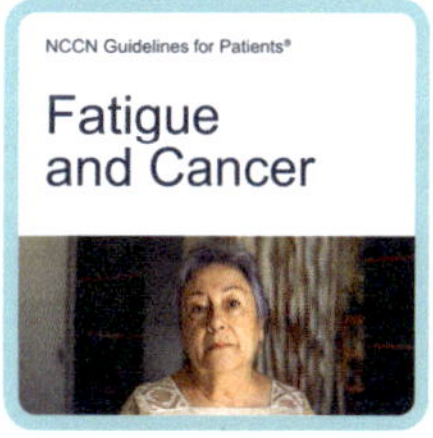

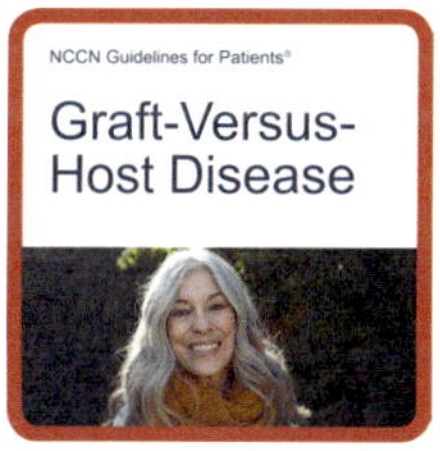

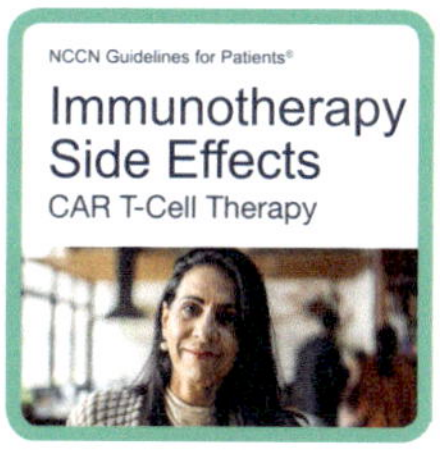

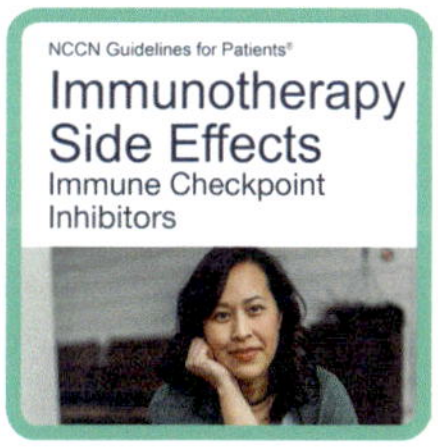

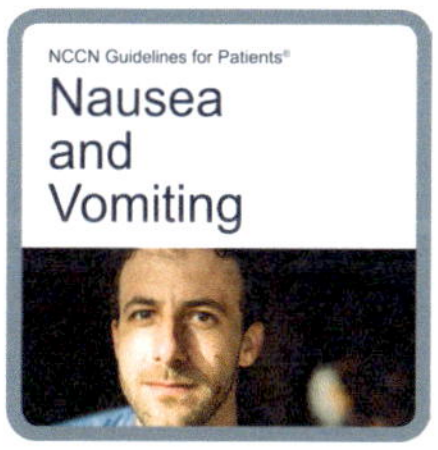

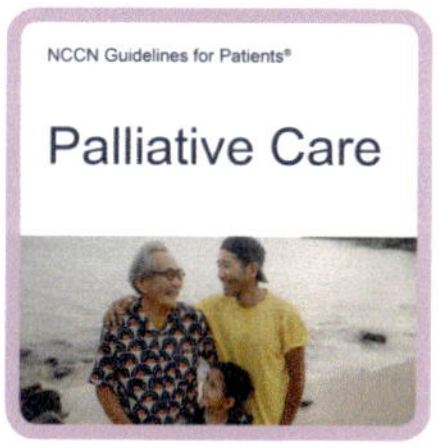

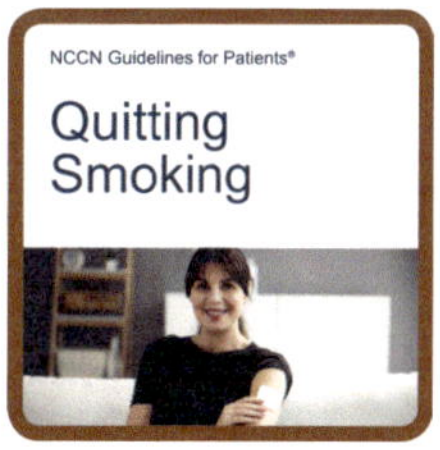

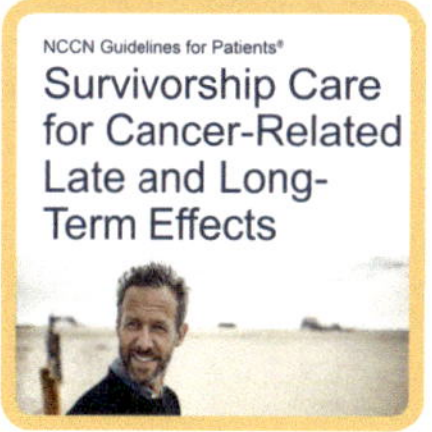

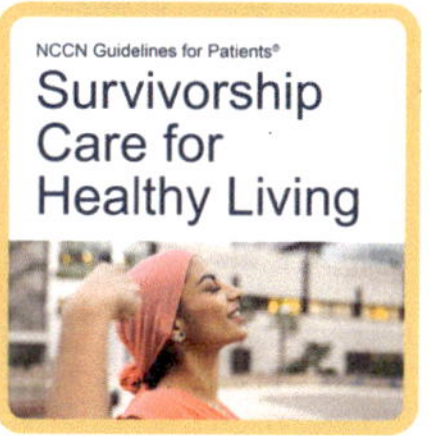

Key points

- WM may return after primary treatment. This is called relapse, and it's common in people with WM.
- Relapsed WM may be treated with the same therapy you had before or with different therapy, depending on your circumstances.
- Sometimes WM can become resistant to treatment, or the effects of treatment don't last very long. People who have WM that's resistant to one treatment can be given a different treatment.
- High-dose chemotherapy with autologous stem cell rescue may be an option for certain people whose WM returns more than once after previous treatments.
- Managing the long-term effects of cancer and its treatment, maintaining your quality of life, and staying connected with family members, friends, and caregivers are important parts of survivorship.
- Supportive care is given at any stage of disease, not just at the end of life.

Questions to ask

- Are you suggesting treatment options from the NCCN Guidelines, or have you modified the treatment approach in my situation?
- What precautions should I know about when choosing further treatment?
- What will happen if I stop treatment?
- What happens if I run out of treatment options?

5
Other resources

Want to learn more? Here's how you can get additional help.

What else to know

This book can help you improve your cancer care. It plainly explains expert recommendations and suggests questions to ask your care team. But it's not the only resource that you have.

You're welcome to receive as much information and help as you need. Many people are interested in learning more about:

- Finding a specialist who is an expert in their cancer
- The side effects from treatment and the treatment for these side effects
- Participating in choosing treatment and in other decisions
- Dealing with WM while coping with other health problems
- Getting financial help

What else to do

Your health care center can help you with next steps. They often have on-site resources to help meet your needs and find answers to your questions. Health care centers can also inform you of resources in your community.

In addition to help from your providers, the resources listed in the section below provide support for people with WM and similar diseases. Look through the list and visit the provided websites to learn more about these organizations.

Where to get help

BMT InfoNet
bmtinfonet.org

Cancer*Care*
cancercare.org

Imerman Angels
imermanangels.org

International Waldenstrom's Macroglobulinemia Foundation
iwmf.com

National Bone Marrow Transplant Link (nbmtLINK)
nbmtlink.org

National Coalition for Cancer Survivorship
canceradvocacy.org

NMDP
nmdp.org

The Leukemia & Lymphoma Society
lls.org/patient-support

Triage Cancer
triagecancer.org

Questions to ask

- Can you recommend a clinical trial I can join?
- How much will treatment cost? How can I find out how much my insurance company will cover?
- Who can I talk to about help with housing, food, and other basic needs?
- What help is available for transportation, childcare, and home care?
- Are there other services available to me and my caregivers?

We want your feedback!

Our goal is to provide helpful and easy-to-understand information on cancer. Take our survey to let us know what we got right and what we could do better.
NCCN.org/patients/feedback

Having cancer is about more than just treatment. Cancer care can be a rollercoaster ride that includes many additional physical and emotional challenges. It's important to know that you can get support for these challenges.

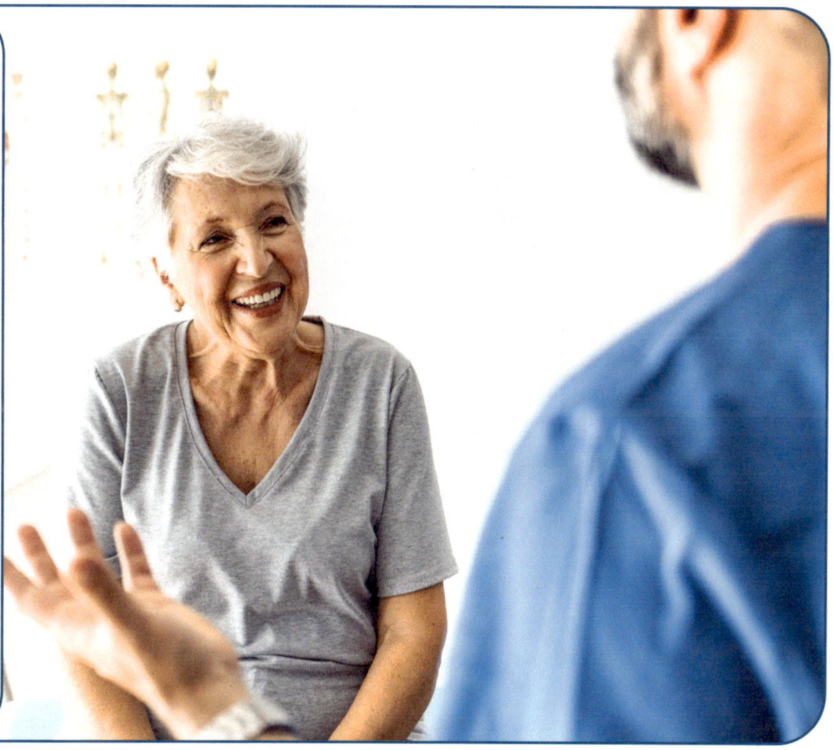

Words to know

amyloidosis
A harmful buildup of an abnormal protein called amyloid.

anemia
A health condition in which the amount of healthy red blood cells is too low to carry enough oxygen to the rest of your body.

antibody
A protein made by white blood cells that helps fight off infection. Also called an immunoglobulin.

B cell
A type of a white blood cell (lymphocyte) that makes antibodies to fight infection.

bone marrow
The soft, sponge-like tissue in the center of most bones where blood cells are made.

bone marrow aspiration
A procedure that removes a liquid bone marrow sample to test for disease.

bone marrow biopsy
A procedure that removes a small amount of solid bone marrow to test for disease.

chemotherapy
A drug treatment that kill fast-growing cells, including cancer cells and normal cells.

clinical trial
A type of research study that analyzes how well investigational tests and drugs work in people.

complete blood count
A blood test that evaluates the number of blood cells in a sample.

hematopathologist
An expert at diagnosing diseases of the blood and bone marrow.

high-dose chemotherapy with autologous stem cell rescue (HDT/ASCR)
A treatment that destroys bone marrow with intense chemotherapy and then restores it with the patient's own healthy stem cells.

hyperviscosity
Abnormally thick blood caused by high levels of immunoglobulin M (IgM).

IgM flare
A temporary increase in IgM level in the blood.

immune system
The body's natural defense against infection and disease.

immunoglobulin
A protein made by white blood cells that helps the body fight off infection. Also called an antibody.

immunoglobulin M (IgM)
The first antibody (immunoglobulin) the immune system makes to fight a new infection. IgM is often found in large amounts in people with WM.

infusion reaction
A bad or overreactive response to an infusion treatment by the immune system.

lymph node
A small, bean-shaped, disease-fighting structure in the immune system.

lymphocyte
A type of immune cell made in the bone marrow and found in blood and in lymph tissue.

lymphoma
Cancer that begins in white blood cells called lymphocytes.

lymphoplasmacytic cells
Cells that have features of both lymphocytes and plasma cells.

lymphoplasmacytic lymphoma (LPL)
A type of lymphoma that starts in the bone marrow and can cause a shortage of blood cells needed by the body. Waldenström macroglobulinemia is the most common form of LPL.

neurologist
An expert in disorders of the nervous system.

peripheral neuropathy
Nerve damage that causes pain, numbness, tingling, burning sensation, swelling, or weakness in parts of the body.

plasma cell
A type of white blood cell that makes large amounts of one type of antibody.

plasma exchange
A procedure that separates and removes plasma from the blood.

progression
The growth or spread of cancer after being tested or treated.

relapse
The return or worsening of cancer after a period of improvement.

shingles
A painful rash that occurs when the virus that causes chickenpox is reactivated in the body.

targeted therapy
The use of medicines that can target and attack cancer cells.

watchful waiting
A period of watching for cancer growth or occurrence while not receiving treatment.

NCCN Contributors

This patient guide is based on the NCCN Clinical Practice Guidelines in Oncology (NCCN Guidelines®) for Waldenström Macroglobulinemia/Lymphoplasmacytic Lymphoma, Version 3.2025. It was adapted, reviewed, and published with help from the following people:

Dorothy A. Shead, MS
Senior Director
Patient Information Operations

John Murphy
Senior Medical Writer

Susan Kidney
Senior Graphic Design Specialist

The NCCN Clinical Practice Guidelines in Oncology (NCCN Guidelines®) for Waldenström Macroglobulinemia/Lymphoplasmacytic Lymphoma, Version 3.2025 were developed by the following NCCN Panel Members:

Shaji K. Kumar, MD
Mayo Clinic Comprehensive Cancer Center

Natalie S. Callander, MD/Vice Chair
University of Wisconsin
Carbone Cancer Center

Kehinde Adekola, MD, MSCI
Robert H. Lurie Comprehensive Cancer Center of Northwestern University

Larry D. Anderson, Jr., MD, PhD
UT Southwestern Simmons Comprehensive Cancer Center

*Muhamed Baljevic, MD
Vanderbilt-Ingram Cancer Center

Rachid Baz, MD
Moffitt Cancer Center

Erica Campagnaro, MD
University of Michigan Rogel Cancer Center

Caitlin Costello, MD
UC San Diego Moores Cancer Center

Christopher D'Angelo, MD
Fred & Pamela Buffett Cancer Center

Benjamin Derman, MD
The UChicago Medicine Comprehensive Cancer Center

*Srinivas Devarakonda, MD
The Ohio State University Comprehensive Cancer Center – James Cancer Hospital and Solove Research Institute

Noura Elsedawy, MD
St. Jude Children's Research Hospital/ The University of Tennessee Health Science Center

*Amandeep Godara, MD
Huntsman Cancer Institute at the University of Utah

Kelly Godby, MD
O'Neal Comprehensive Cancer Center at UAB

Jens Hillengass, MD, PhD
Roswell Park Comprehensive Cancer Center

Leona Holmberg, MD, PhD
Fred Hutchinson Cancer Center

Myo Htut, MD
City of Hope National Medical Center

Carol Ann Huff, MD
Johns Hopkins Kimmel Cancer Center

Malin Hultcrantz, MD, PhD
Memorial Sloan Kettering Cancer Center

Yubin Kang, MD
Duke Cancer Institute

Sarah Larson, MD
UCLA Jonsson Comprehensive Cancer Center

Hans C. Lee, MD
The University of Texas MD Anderson Cancer Center

Michaela Liedtke, MD
Stanford Cancer Institute

Thomas Martin, MD
UCSF Helen Diller Family Comprehensive Cancer Center

James Omel, MD
Patient Advocate

Timothy Robinson, MD, PhD
Yale Cancer Center/Smilow Cancer Hospital

Aaron Rosenberg, MD
UC Davis Comprehensive Cancer Center

*Shayna R. Sarosiek, MD
Dana-Farber/Brigham and Women's Cancer Center

Mark A. Schroeder, MD
Siteman Cancer Center at Barnes-Jewish Hospital and Washington University School of Medicine

Daniel Sherbenou, MD, PhD
University of Colorado Cancer Center

Attaya Suvannasankha, MD
Indiana University Melvin and Bren Simon Comprehensive Cancer Center

Jason Valent, MD
Case Comprehensive Cancer Center/ University Hospitals Seidman Cancer Center and Cleveland Clinic Taussig Cancer Institute

Asya Nina Varshavsky-Yanovsky, MD, PhD
Fox Chase Cancer Center

Dan Vogl, MD
Abramson Cancer Center at the University of Pennsylvania

NCCN

Emily Kovach
Guidelines Layout Specialist

Rashmi Kumar, PhD
Senior Director, Clinical Content

Megan Lyons, MS
Associate Scientist/Medical Writer

* Reviewed this patient guide. For disclosures, visit NCCN.org/disclosures.

NCCN Cancer Centers

Abramson Cancer Center
at the University of Pennsylvania
Philadelphia, Pennsylvania
800.789.7366 • pennmedicine.org/cancer

Case Comprehensive Cancer Center/
University Hospitals Seidman Cancer Center and
Cleveland Clinic Taussig Cancer Institute
Cleveland, Ohio
UH Seidman Cancer Center
800.641.2422 • uhhospitals.org/services/cancer-services
CC Taussig Cancer Institute
866.223.8100 • my.clevelandclinic.org/departments/cancer
Case CCC
216.844.8797 • case.edu/cancer

City of Hope National Medical Center
Duarte, California
800.826.4673 • cityofhope.org

Dana-Farber/Brigham and Women's Cancer Center |
Mass General Cancer Center
Boston, Massachusetts
877.442.3324 • youhaveus.org
617.726.5130 • massgeneral.org/cancer-center

Duke Cancer Institute
Durham, North Carolina
888.275.3853 • dukecancerinstitute.org

Fox Chase Cancer Center
Philadelphia, Pennsylvania
888.369.2427 • foxchase.org

Fred & Pamela Buffett Cancer Center
Omaha, Nebraska
402.559.5600 • unmc.edu/cancercenter

Fred Hutchinson Cancer Center
Seattle, Washington
206.667.5000 • fredhutch.org

Huntsman Cancer Institute at the University of Utah
Salt Lake City, Utah
800.824.2073 • healthcare.utah.edu/huntsmancancerinstitute

Indiana University Melvin and Bren Simon
Comprehensive Cancer Center
Indianapolis, Indiana
888.600.4822 • www.cancer.iu.edu

Johns Hopkins Kimmel Cancer Center
Baltimore, Maryland
410.955.8964
www.hopkinskimmelcancercenter.org

Mayo Clinic Comprehensive Cancer Center
Phoenix/Scottsdale, Arizona
Jacksonville, Florida
Rochester, Minnesota
480.301.8000 • Arizona
904.953.0853 • Florida
507.538.3270 • Minnesota
mayoclinic.org/cancercenter

Memorial Sloan Kettering Cancer Center
New York, New York
800.525.2225 • mskcc.org

Moffitt Cancer Center
Tampa, Florida
888.663.3488 • moffitt.org

O'Neal Comprehensive Cancer Center at UAB
Birmingham, Alabama
800.822.0933 • uab.edu/onealcancercenter

Robert H. Lurie Comprehensive Cancer Center
of Northwestern University
Chicago, Illinois
866.587.4322 • cancer.northwestern.edu

Roswell Park Comprehensive Cancer Center
Buffalo, New York
877.275.7724 • roswellpark.org

Siteman Cancer Center at Barnes-Jewish Hospital
and Washington University School of Medicine
St. Louis, Missouri
800.600.3606 • siteman.wustl.edu

St. Jude Children's Research Hospital/
The University of Tennessee Health Science Center
Memphis, Tennessee
866.278.5833 • stjude.org
901.448.5500 • uthsc.edu

Stanford Cancer Institute
Stanford, California
877.668.7535 • cancer.stanford.edu

The Ohio State University Comprehensive Cancer Center -
James Cancer Hospital and Solove Research Institute
Columbus, Ohio
800.293.5066 • cancer.osu.edu

The UChicago Medicine Comprehensive Cancer Center
Chicago, Illinois
773.702.1000 • uchicagomedicine.org/cancer

The University of Texas MD Anderson Cancer Center
Houston, Texas
844.269.5922 • mdanderson.org

UC Davis Comprehensive Cancer Center
Sacramento, California
916.734.5959 • 800.770.9261
health.ucdavis.edu/cancer

UC San Diego Moores Cancer Center
La Jolla, California
858.822.6100 • cancer.ucsd.edu

UCLA Jonsson Comprehensive Cancer Center
Los Angeles, California
310.825.5268 • uclahealth.org/cancer

UCSF Helen Diller Family
Comprehensive Cancer Center
San Francisco, California
800.689.8273 • cancer.ucsf.edu

University of Colorado Cancer Center
Aurora, Colorado
720.848.0300 • coloradocancercenter.org

University of Michigan Rogel Cancer Center
Ann Arbor, Michigan
800.865.1125 • rogelcancercenter.org

University of Wisconsin Carbone Cancer Center
Madison, Wisconsin
608.265.1700 • uwhealth.org/cancer

UT Southwestern Simmons
Comprehensive Cancer Center
Dallas, Texas
214.648.3111 • utsouthwestern.edu/simmons

Vanderbilt-Ingram Cancer Center
Nashville, Tennessee
877.936.8422 • vicc.org

Yale Cancer Center/Smilow Cancer Hospital
New Haven, Connecticut
855.4.SMILOW • yalecancercenter.org

share with us.

Take our survey and help make the NCCN Guidelines for Patients better for everyone!

NCCN.org/patients/comments

Index

Made in the USA
Monee, IL
05 November 2026

67380075R00031